EFT Tapping for Weight Loss

A Women's 3-Week Beginner Step-by-Step Guide with Sample EFT Tapping Scripts

STEPHANIE HINDEROCK

Disclaimer

By reading this disclaimer, you are accepting the terms of the disclaimer in full. If you disagree with this disclaimer, please do not read the guide.

All of the content within this guide is provided for informational and educational purposes only, and should not be accepted as independent medical or other professional advice. The author is not a doctor, physician, nurse, mental health provider, or registered nutritionist/dietician. Therefore, using and reading this guide does not establish any form of a physician-patient relationship.

Always consult with a physician or another qualified health provider with any issues or questions you might have regarding any sort of medical condition. Do not ever disregard any qualified professional medical advice or delay seeking that advice because of anything you have read in this guide. The information in this guide is not intended to be any sort of medical advice and should not be used in lieu of any medical advice by a licensed and qualified medical professional.

The information in this guide has been compiled from a variety of known sources. However, the author cannot attest to or guarantee the accuracy of each source and thus should not be held liable for any errors or omissions.

You acknowledge that the publisher of this guide will not be held liable for any loss or damage of any kind incurred as a result of this guide or the reliance on any information provided within this guide. You acknowledge and agree that you assume all risk and responsibility for any action you undertake in response to the information in this guide.

Using this guide does not guarantee any particular result (e.g., weight loss or a cure). By reading this guide, you acknowledge that there are no guarantees to any specific outcome or results you can expect.

All product names, diet plans, or names used in this guide are for identification purposes only and are the property of their respective owners. The use of these names does not imply endorsement. All other trademarks cited herein are the property of their respective owners.

Where applicable, this guide is not intended to be a substitute for the original work of this diet plan and is, at most, a supplement to the original work for this diet plan and never a direct substitute. This guide is a personal expression of the facts of that diet plan.

Where applicable, persons shown in the cover images are stock photography models and the publisher has obtained the rights to use the images through license agreements with third-party stock image companies.

Introduction

Have you ever had trouble losing weight no matter how hard you restricted your calorie intake, or how vigorously you exercised daily? We know we have had our fair share of frustrating experiences here and there. If you're just like many other women out there, you know how it feels to practically exhaust all efforts to no avail.

While this may be very troubling and may seem like a hopeless feat, you might take comfort in knowing that you aren't alone. In the years 2017 and 2018, the recorded percentage of people suffering from obesity in the United States alone was a whopping 42.4%, and those who suffered from severe obesity comprised 9.2% of the population.

This, however, should be taken seriously as obesity in itself is serious and costly regardless of how prevalent it may be. Imagine just how many people are free from obesity, but suffer from weight problems nevertheless.

If you're looking for a good solution to your weight problems, obese or not, and would like to find a safe, non-invasive way to get rid of your stubborn fat, or simply just shed a few pounds, there's an alternative method that's available on the market as we speak.

EFT Tapping, or emotional freedom technique, is a good way for you to address not only your weight problems but has great benefits on your mental health, as well.

In this 3-week guide for EFT Tapping, these are going to be your basic takeaways:

- Discover the benefits of keeping yourself not only physically, but mentally, fit regularly;
- Learn to channel balanced energy levels for overall health;
- Discover important pressure points to address specific problems in addition to weight loss;
- Adopt a weight loss regimen that best suits you;
- Learn to sustain EFT Tapping even after the end of the program.

Table of Contents

WHAT IS EFT TAPPING?

EFT tapping, also known as Emotional Freedom Technique, is a form of alternative therapy that involves tapping on specific points in the body to release negative emotions and promote healing. This technique is based on the idea that emotional stress can cause physical symptoms and by tapping on certain acupuncture points, energy blockages can be released.

This is a form of therapy that can be used to treat physical pain, mental health issues, addictions, and even weight loss.

EFT tapping was developed by Gary Craig and has been around since the 1990s. It has gained more popularity in recent years due to its effectiveness in treating a variety of different conditions.

Use Cases of EFT Tapping

EFT tapping can be used to treat many different conditions, including:

1. Weight loss: EFT tapping can help with weight loss by addressing the emotional and psychological factors that contribute to overeating or unhealthy eating habits. By

tapping on specific acupressure points while focusing on negative emotions related to food cravings or body image issues, individuals may experience a reduction in these feelings and therefore be less likely to turn to food as a coping mechanism.

2. Anxiety and stress management: EFT tapping is effective in reducing symptoms of anxiety and stress by calming the nervous system and promoting relaxation. Through tapping on certain acupressure points while acknowledging negative thoughts or emotions, individuals may experience a decrease in their intensity, leading to a greater sense of calm.

3. Pain relief: EFT tapping can also help manage pain by targeting the underlying emotional causes of physical discomfort. By using tapping techniques alongside affirmations focused on acceptance and self-compassion, individuals may experience a reduction in pain levels.

4. Trauma recovery: EFT tapping has been used as part of trauma-focused therapy to help individuals process traumatic memories and emotions in a safe and supportive environment. By combining tapping with guided visualization or other therapeutic techniques, individuals may find relief from symptoms related to PTSD or other trauma-related disorders.

Overall, EFT tapping is thought to work by stimulating the body's natural healing processes through a combination of acupressure point stimulation and cognitive-behavioral techniques. While it may not work for everyone, many people have reported positive benefits from incorporating EFT into their self-care routine.

Why is it important to Lose Weight?

Weight loss is important for a variety of reasons. Not only can it improve physical health, but it can also help with mental and emotional well-being.

Here are some reasons why it is important to lose weight:

1. **Decreased Risk of Chronic Diseases** - Your body weight can have a drastic effect on your risk of chronic diseases. In recent years, numerous studies have highlighted the importance of maintaining a healthy weight to significantly decrease the risk of diseases such as diabetes, heart disease, and stroke. All it takes is a loss of 5-10% of your total body weight for an impactful reduction - any smaller than that can be ineffective.

2. **Improved Sleep Quality** - When excess weight is present, this increases one's risk of developing sleep apnea and other breathing difficulties. Losing weight will enable you to sleep better, and once this is achieved it can make a world of difference in terms of energy during the day. Those who feel rested and energized are more likely to achieve the goals they set out for themselves - whether physical or mental. Therefore, investing in one's health through weight loss can be an invaluable decision that pays off substantially over time.

3. **Increased Energy Levels** - Consuming fewer calories and losing weight can help an individual boost their energy levels. When an individual has less body mass, they require less energy to move around, allowing them

to do more throughout the day. Moreover, lowering their fat intake and improving blood sugar control helps improve an individual's energy, as it lowers the surges and dips in blood sugar that can cause fatigue and lethargy.

4. **Enhanced Mood** - Reducing excess weight has been shown to have a positive effect on mental well-being. As the body sheds extra pounds, self-confidence can cultivate through improved body image and a decrease in medical issues that impact the body. It is increasingly evident that the link between depression and anxiety can be minimized or eradicated simply by shedding a few pounds. Studies show that losing weight brings about an overall improvement in mood, reducing stress levels and making life more enjoyable.

5. **Better Joint Health** - Maintaining a healthy weight is an important part of better joint health. Individuals who are overweight experience extra stress on their joints, including the knees and hips. This pressure is the result of carrying too much body mass, which exacerbates joint issues and increases wear and tear over time. Fortunately, losing excess weight can help to reduce this strain, thereby alleviating joint discomfort and preserving joint integrity for longer periods. All in all, managing body weight is an effective way to promote better joint health.

6. **Improved Digestion** - Shedding excess weight is one tactic that can be used to improve digestive health. Extra pounds can put increased pressure on vital organs, particularly the digestive tract, leading to uncomfortable and sometimes painful issues such as

acid reflux and bloating. Weight loss acts to reduce this strain by lessening the amount of force being applied. This often results in improved digestion, enabling more effective absorption of essential nutrients from food. Therefore, those suffering from digestive ailments would be well-served by making an effort to reduce their weight to attain a healthier digestive system.

7. **Lowered Blood Pressure** - High blood pressure is an important yet often neglected risk factor when it comes to heart health. Elevated blood pressure can cause damage to the blood vessels, heart, and organs throughout the body, causing potentially serious complications such as heart attack and stroke. Fortunately, studies have demonstrated that achieving even a modest weight loss is associated with lower blood pressure levels in hypertensive individuals.

8. **Reduced Risk of Cancer** - Obesity is a significant risk factor associated with many types of cancer, including breast, colon, kidney, liver, ovarian, pancreatic, and uterine. The risk of these cancers can be significantly reduced by maintaining a healthy weight through regular exercise and a balanced diet. Although a certain amount of risk cannot be eliminated no matter the lifestyle changes, being able to control obesity does provide valuable protection against many types of cancer.

9. **Increased Longevity** - Studies have given us better insight into whether being overweight or obese can contribute to an earlier death than those who maintain a healthy body mass index (BMI). It has been found that a person's life expectancy can span further through care and consideration of their health. For those looking to

add years to their lifespan, it is best practice to keep the BMI within recommended ranges.

10. **Improved Overall Quality of Life** - The health effects of excess pounds extend to areas beyond physical appearance and can be far-reaching both emotionally and physically. When a person finds success in losing excess weight, their physical health improves in terms of energy levels, fat composition, muscles, and joints. Additionally, increasing the metabolic rate helps to regulate moods more effectively due to better blood oxygenation. Furthermore, foods that are easier to digest are often recommended as part of an effective weight loss plan which leads to improved overall digestion. Thus, it is clear that by improving these key aspects of bodily health, people often find themselves with a greatly improved overall quality of life after losing excess pounds.

EFT Tapping for Weight Loss

The emotional freedom technique, or EFT, is considered an alternative treatment that doesn't involve the use of conventional medicine or healing techniques to address both physical and emotional distress and pain. Some people may know this simply as psychological acupressure, or tapping.

According to Gary Craig, its developer, tapping on certain parts of the body, known as pressure points, can help you balance your inner energy and reduce both forms of pain. It, therefore, provides an easy way to receive treatment, and some may even be able to treat themselves if the technique is properly taught.

Practitioners say that its most common usage is for anxiety and post-traumatic stress disorder (PTSD) treatment; however, EFT tapping has also been observed to have some positive benefits on weight.

Most weight loss programs and exercise regimens require you to restrict caloric intake to attain a deficit and work out at least 5 days a week throughout the program. While this may be good for short-term weight loss, this doesn't necessarily ensure longevity.

Most programs that cater to women's needs promise hourglass figures by the end of the fixed term, without necessarily considering different body types and metabolic rates, and while the advertising sounds quite promising, the results may end up disappointing instead.

Unlike these, EFT Tapping addresses the root causes of your weight gain and/or stubborn weight. By pinpointing the exact reason and area concerned, Tapping can subsequently be used to shed those extra pounds and keep them off, resulting in sustained weight loss or weight maintenance which, as mentioned, most — if not all — exercise and weight loss programs don't offer. Unless they advise you to stay on the program for good, then the results you get with those are only good so long as you're still actually on them.

The different points used in EFT tapping

The important parts of your body to take note of, or the meridian points involved in EFT Tapping are as follows:

The top of your head or the "Hundred Meeting Points" Meridian: This location, which may also be referred to as the Hundred Meeting Points, can be found at the very top of the head. When this meridian is activated, a person can tap into their inner wisdom, which provides them with insights and clarity. A person's spiritual connection can also be opened up with this practice, and any harsh critiques they may have directed on themselves as a result of their inability to concentrate successfully can be eliminated as a side benefit. EFT-tapping users can acquire increased mindfulness in their daily lives by unleashing their real potential through this potent meridian point once the pressure associated with this point has been released.

The side of your eye, or the Gall Bladder Meridian: An excellent way for treating a wide range of emotional difficulties is to apply pressure on the side of the eye at the Meridian Point, which is also referred to as the Gall Bladder Meridian. It is possible to get insight into challenging feelings like hate and anger using the EFT Tapping technique. In addition to this, it helps to expand one's understanding as well as their capacity for compassion.

The eyebrow, or the Bladder Meridian: A potent acupressure point that can bring about emotional healing and inner serenity is located between the eyebrows. In traditional Chinese medicine, this point is also referred to as the Bladder Meridian. It is said that stimulating this area can remove feelings of trauma, melancholy, emotional anguish or hurt, impatience, restlessness, and irritation.

Those who focus their attention on this particular meridian may discover that they experience a sense of release from negative emotions and find that they are more suited to deal with the stresses that they encounter in their day-to-day life. It's possible that incorporating acupressure techniques into your self-care regimen might be an efficient approach to boost both your mental and physical health, so keep that in mind as you read on.

The under eye, or the Stomach Meridian: A potent acupressure point that may bring forth feelings of contentment, safety, and peace is located just beneath the eye, and this area is also referred to as the Stomach Meridian. This point, when stimulated, can assist ease feelings of dread, concern, anxiety, disappointment, and emptiness. It is located on the upper part of the back, between the shoulder blades.

When individuals consistently apply a light amount of pressure to this spot, they can find respite from the emotional tensions in their lives and gain a stronger feeling of inner peace. Activating the under-eye point can be a straightforward and efficient method of fostering overall well-being as well as emotional equilibrium. This can be accomplished through acupuncture or acupressure treatments.

Under your nose or the Governing Meridian: Within the realm of traditional Chinese medicine, the Governing Meridian, which is often referred to as "Under your nose," is a potent method for fostering feelings of self-affirmation, self-empowerment, and acceptance. People can let go of unpleasant feelings such as shame, guilt, humiliation, impotence, fear of failure, and sadness when they work with this meridian. Instead, they should work on developing compassion for both themselves and the others around them.

This method encourages individuals to feel more confident and capable in their day-to-day lives while also cultivating a positive mentality that supports emotional well-being. It is also helpful in reducing feelings of anxiety and depression. Explore the advantages of the Governing Meridian now if you want to increase your emotional fortitude and a general feeling of self-worth, and consider doing so if you are wanting to strengthen your emotional resilience.

The chin, or the Central Meridian: In traditional Chinese medicine, the chin is referred to as the Central Meridian. This is because it is thought to contain key energy points that affect an individual's emotional and mental condition. It is stated that by stimulating this region, a person might experience clarity, self-acceptance, confidence, and a sense of absolute assurance.

On the other side, ignoring this aspect might result in a state of doubt, bewilderment, humiliation, and embarrassment for the individual. When we take care of our chins by giving them frequent massages or using acupressure points, we may help clear any blockages that may be present in this area and support the flow of positive energy throughout the body.

The collarbone, or the Kidney Meridian: It is claimed that the collarbone, which in traditional Chinese medicine is also referred to as the Kidney Meridian, has major energy points that affect an individual's emotional and mental condition. Stimulating this region helps foster confidence, clarity, and fluidity in one's pursuit of objectives and ambitions, which can all help go forward.

It has been suggested that ignoring this region may result in a lack of decisiveness, anxiety, stagnancy, and tension. We may clear any blockages in this meridian and encourage good energy flow throughout the body if we take care of our collarbone by giving it frequent massages or using acupressure. This can assist us in overcoming barriers and problems that may have been preventing us from realizing our full potential up until now.

The underarm, or the Spleen Meridian: The underarm, which is also referred to as the Spleen Meridian, is a significant energy channel in the body that has a significant influence on the state of our mental and emotional health. This meridian, when stimulated, has the potential to bring forth feelings of clarity, calm, confidence, and compassion toward oneself as well as others.

It can remove unfavorable feelings such as anxiety, guilt, hopelessness, poor self-esteem, and insecurity from one's life. We can liberate the power of this region of the body to bring about internal harmony and balance when we concentrate our attention on it by utilizing methods such as acupressure and acupuncture.

Karate chop point: A strong acupressure method for eliminating bad emotions and fostering happy sentiments, the Karate chop point is located on the upper back, between the shoulder blades. Individuals may swiftly and simply dissolve any emotional obstacles that may be holding them back from reaching their objectives by applying light pressure to the outside border of the hand. This technique is also known as the "hand release." This strategy has the potential to make us feel more at ease, more focused, and better prepared to meet any obstacle that may come our way.

During an EFT session, you will tap each point while reciting particular words relating to weight loss and any emotions or concerns around it that you wish to address. These phrases can be tailored to target a specific issue or emotion. The particular wording will change depending on what it is that you are working on directly, but it may be something along the lines of "Even though I struggle with my weight, I love and accept myself fully and totally."

HOW CAN EFT TAPPING HELP WITH WEIGHT LOSS?

When you first begin your journey to weight loss, you might think that all you have to do is attain a caloric deficit to shed those extra pounds and follow a strict diet thereafter to maintain it. While this may be true, diets may lead to adverse effects in the long run, especially when you follow a diet that cuts certain food groups off, and ultimately, certain nutrients that you can only get from those foods. Aside from this, the more restrictive your diet gets, the more likely you are to be susceptible to cravings and, for most, binge eating.

Women, in particular, are quite conscious when it comes to their weight, and this can have drastic adverse effects on their self-image and confidence. This is the reason why fad diets and diets, in general, have been created, with women as the target market.

What you have to understand before anything else is that EFT Tapping is not a form of diet. It's something to be incorporated into your lifestyle, and although it may seem negligible at first, it can lead to great results that you could both see and feel in the long run. Most practitioners can attest to its effectiveness, and once you learn the ropes, you will, too.

EFT Tapping addresses certain issues by first dealing with its mental aspects. This is something unique about this method, as most of the diets offered in general don't pay enough attention to how you feel about yourself, but focus largely on how you want to look at the end of the day. EFT Tapping, however, acknowledges the impact of your emotions on your overall physique, as your emotions are, simply put, the basis of your actions which lead to the results you produce and what you make of the situation and yourself.

Stress, Negative Emotions, and Weight Gain

Stress and negative emotions can have a significant impact on our physical health, including contributing to weight gain. When we experience stress or negative emotions, our bodies release cortisol, a hormone that can increase appetite and cause us to store fat in certain areas of the body.

One way that stress can contribute to weight gain is through emotional eating. Many people turn to food as a way to cope with stress or negative emotions, which can lead to overeating and consuming more calories than our bodies need. This is because when we eat high-fat or high-sugar foods, our brains release dopamine, which can create feelings of pleasure and temporarily reduce feelings of stress or anxiety.

Another way that stress can contribute to weight gain is through disrupted sleep patterns. When we are stressed or anxious, it can be difficult to fall asleep or stay asleep throughout the night. This lack of restful sleep can disrupt the hormonal balance in our bodies and increase levels of cortisol, leading to increased appetite and weight gain.

Stress also affects the digestive system by slowing down digestion and causing inflammation in the gut. This inflammation can lead to bloating and discomfort, making it difficult for our bodies to properly digest and absorb nutrients from food. As a result, we may feel hungrier than usual even after eating a full meal.

Negative emotions such as sadness or depression can also contribute to weight gain by reducing motivation for physical activity and healthy eating habits. When we feel down or depressed, it can be challenging to find the energy or desire to exercise regularly or prepare healthy meals at home. Instead, we may turn to comfort foods that are high in calories but low in nutritional value.

In addition, negative emotions like anxiety or low self-esteem can lead to binge eating behaviors where individuals consume large amounts of food in one sitting without feeling satisfied. Binge eating often leads individuals to feel guilty and ashamed about their behavior which further perpetuates unhealthy behaviors around food.

Albert Bandura's theory of self-efficacy

The self-efficacy theory developed by Albert Bandura is a strong tool that can assist individuals in accomplishing their objectives regarding weight loss. Individuals are more likely to remain motivated, make healthy choices, and avoid emotional eating induced by stress or negative emotions if they believe in their capacity to accomplish tasks and achieve objectives. Believing in one's ability to complete tasks and achieve goals is essential.

According to self-efficacy theory, an individual's ideas about their potential to achieve are shaped by four different types of information: experiences of mastery, vicarious experiences, social persuasion, and physiological and emotional states. Experiences of mastery entail effectively accomplishing tasks, which boosts one's sense of their efficacy. Increasing one's sense of self-efficacy may be accomplished through the use of vicarious experiences, which consist of witnessing other people completing tasks.

Receiving positive feedback or encouragement from others, which can lead to an increased sense of self-efficacy, is an essential component of social persuasion. Physiological and affective states, on the other hand, allude to how a person's physical and emotional condition might influence the belief that they have in their abilities.

The self-efficacy hypothesis, when applied to the topic of weight reduction, proposes that having a sense of confidence in one's capacity to reduce weight is one of the most important factors in achieving success. Having conviction in oneself helps individuals stay motivated through the ups and downs of the path toward weight loss, while also supporting healthy eating choices and frequent exercise.

Emotional Freedom Technique (EFT) Tapping for Weight Loss is One Approach That Builds On the Foundation of Bandura's Theory As was noted earlier, EFT Tapping is a sort of psychological acupressure that includes focusing on limiting beliefs or unpleasant emotions while tapping on certain energy meridian points. Individuals can reduce the triggers for emotional eating and develop a greater sense of control over their food choices if they tap away negative emotions such as stress or anxiety related to food or body image issues. This can be accomplished by tapping away negative emotions such as stress or anxiety.

EFT Tapping for weight loss combines the ideas of Bandura's theory by enhancing self-efficacy through the use of positive affirmations during tapping sessions. This is in addition to minimizing emotional eating triggers, which is the primary goal of EFT Tapping for weight loss. These affirmations are meant to help people feel more confident in their abilities to make healthy decisions about their diet and their level of physical activity.

When taken as a whole, implementing Bandura's theory of self-efficacy through techniques such as EFT Tapping for weight reduction might assist individuals in overcoming roadblocks along the path toward accomplishing their desired level of weight loss. It is much simpler to maintain one's motivation when they have built up a solid feeling of self-confidence in their capabilities, which also makes it easier to make good choices.

How EFT Tapping Can Help Women Lose Weight

As repeatedly emphasized in the previous chapters, the correlation between EFT Tapping and weight loss is quite simple: it delves into the emotional and mental aspects of your overall health, instead of merely focusing on what's on the outside.

Because EMT Tapping aims and is designed to lower anxiety levels by tapping one of eight parts of your body called or referred to as energy meridians by practitioners, you are lowering your stress levels and boosting your confidence. Once the energy balance is brought back, you become more aware of your eating habits and thus become a significant factor in weight loss.

If it doesn't make that much sense to you yet, here's a thorough breakdown of why EFT Tapping and reducing stress levels can be an effective weight loss mechanism. Studies show that there is a correlation between stress and the tendency to overeat and, ultimately, weight gain.

Most people call this "emotional eating" or "stress eating", and the reason why this happens is because of the release of cortisol that takes place when stress is being built up, and this then leads to increased appetite. The most important factor that has been accounted for in weight gain is, therefore, the psychological state of the person.

The same study also shows that these extreme cortisol levels derived from emotional distress can also affect your cravings for fatty, sugary, and generally unhealthy foods.

Women in particular are more susceptible to this because of a hormonal imbalance involving estrogen and serotonin that can lead to food cravings, especially when it comes to comfort foods. The constantly fluctuating hormones caused by women's menstrual cycles are the biggest culprit in this regard. Pregnant women in particular tend to experience these cravings at extreme levels because of hormonal changes.

By lowering stress levels, therefore, you get balanced cortisol levels and thereby prevent any chances of binge eating, emotional eating, or stress eating. There is then increased awareness of what you do, and how you eat, and it's an overall healthier coping mechanism that can steer you clear of those extra pounds. EFT Tapping addresses this specifically by activating your amygdala, thus regulating any fear and anxiety that may be welling up.

The Advantages of EFT Tapping for Weight Loss

EFT Tapping is a unique and effective technique that offers several advantages over other weight loss programs, including its ability to reduce stress, address emotional eating, promote mind-body connection, ease of learning, and lack of side effects or risks associated with its use.

Here are some of the advantages of EFT Tapping for weight loss:

1. Reduces Stress: EFT Tapping is a technique that involves tapping on specific acupressure points while focusing on negative emotions and feelings. This process has been shown to reduce stress levels, which can be a major contributor to overeating and weight gain. By reducing stress, EFT Tapping can help individuals make healthier choices when it comes to food and exercise.

2. Addresses Emotional Eating: Emotional eating is a common issue for many people struggling with weight loss. EFT Tapping can help address the underlying emotional issues that may be causing individuals to turn to food for comfort or as a coping mechanism. By

addressing these emotional triggers, individuals may be better able to control their eating habits and make healthier choices.

3. Promotes Mind-Body Connection: EFT Tapping promotes the connection between the mind and body, allowing individuals to become more aware of their thoughts and emotions about their weight loss journey. This awareness can lead to increased self-control and motivation when it comes to making healthy choices.

4. Easy to Learn: Unlike many other weight loss programs that require extensive training or knowledge, EFT Tapping is easy to learn and can be done at home without any special equipment or resources. This accessibility makes it an ideal option for those who may not have the time or resources for other weight loss programs.

5. No Side Effects: Unlike some weight loss medications or supplements, EFT Tapping has no known side effects or risks associated with its use. This makes it a safe option for those who may have health concerns or sensitivities to certain medications.

6. Sustainable: EFT Tapping is a sustainable weight loss solution because it focuses on addressing the root cause of weight gain instead of just treating the symptoms. By addressing emotional triggers and promoting self-awareness, individuals can develop long-term healthy habits that will help them maintain their weight loss goals.

7. Cost-Effective: Compared to other weight loss programs or treatments, EFT Tapping is a cost-effective option. There are no ongoing costs or fees

associated with its use, making it an affordable option for those on a budget.

8. Individualized Approach: EFT Tapping is an individualized approach to weight loss that takes into account each person's unique emotional needs and triggers. This personalized approach can lead to better results than a one-size-fits-all approach.

9. Can be Used in Conjunction with Other Programs: EFT Tapping can be used in conjunction with other weight loss programs or treatments, such as diet and exercise plans, to enhance their effectiveness. This makes it a versatile option for those looking to boost their weight loss efforts.

10. Improves Overall Well-Being: In addition to helping with weight loss, EFT Tapping has been shown to improve overall well-being by reducing stress levels and promoting relaxation. This can lead to improved mental health, better sleep quality, and increased energy levels - all of which can contribute to successful weight loss outcomes.

WHAT YOU SHOULD KNOW BEFORE TRYING EFT TAPPING

A few things that you should know about EFT Tapping are: (1) the practice of Tapping doesn't carry with it any side effects, and is completely safe to try; however, this may not be the best weight loss solution for those who suffer from an obsessive-compulsive disorder or OCD, as it may form part of your compulsive behavior; and (2) for those who intend to practice EFT Tapping to address any mental health issues or conditions, it would be best to consult a mental health professional before trying it out yourself.

Once you've decided to begin practicing EFT Tapping, it is highly recommended to first come up with affirmation statements that could help you stay on track and keep yourself feeling empowered, as well as remind you of your goals. In this specific instance, if EFT Tapping is something you'd like to start practicing for weight loss, it's highly suggested to have an affirmation statement regarding body positivity and self-confidence. This can be used not only during Tapping but also during those times when you feel inclined to give in to your cravings or food temptations.

The meridian points to keep in mind when Tapping for weight loss are the following:

- The area between your index finger and thumb, or the karate chop;
- Chin;
- Underarm;
- The outer part of the eye;
- Under the eye;
- Eyebrows;
- Under the nose; and
- Inner point of the collarbone.

For optimum results, EFT Tapping may be practiced in addition to other activities such as yoga, pilates, and high-intensity interval training.

BEGINNING YOUR PROGRAM — WEEK 1

For the first week, you can ease into the program by coming up with an affirmation statement involving and addressing your confidence level. Something along the lines of "although I don't think I can pull this off, I know what I'm capable of and I can certainly do this" could be a good start.

While repeating your affirmation statement, slowly start taking deep breaths in and deep breaths out, slowly. Then initiate your Tapping by tapping the area right outside of your eyes gently.

Repeat this thrice, and remember: while you are breathing, you are taking in positive energy, and getting rid of negative energy.

Continue tapping repeatedly, and recite your affirmation statement internally: I know I haven't been the best version of myself, but I'm positive I'll get my confidence back. This is what I deserve.

Deep breaths again; positivity in, negativity out. Release the tension, and start tapping again.

Affirm yourself once more: I deserve the best. I deserve love, and above all, I deserve to love myself. I will win this fight by reaching my goals. I will boost my self-esteem. I will feel better about myself, this I'm sure of.

Move on to a different meridian point and repeat the following statements while doing so:

- Under your eyes – I will stay focused on my goal.
- At the top of my head – I will remember why I started.
- Inner point of your collarbone – I will love myself more.

Lastly, return to the starting point, which is the outer part of your eyes, and take deep breaths in, and deep breaths out.

STRENGTHENING YOUR SENSE OF SELF – WEEK 2

Now, for the second week, your affirmation statement should involve the reinforcement of how you felt or wanted to feel during the first week to keep you going.

Around this time, you should be feeling a stronger sense of self from the Tapping exercises you completed the previous week; if not, that isn't a problem at all. Just keep going, and stay focused. The stress and emotional baggage will slowly start to disappear, along with your cravings, if done consistently.

Remind yourself by saying something along the lines of, "I'm already on this journey, and I know I can stick with it and see it through until the end".

Take deep breaths in, and focus on letting the positive energy enter. Then take deep breaths, and do away with the negative energy.

Tap the top of your head, and recite to yourself your affirmation statement. I now have more confidence in my ability to see this through. I am now more certain that I can do this. I am stronger than I think.

Repeat the same sequence as the first week, and shift your attention to the fact that you're already halfway through the program, and your consistency is helping you get there, even though you initially thought you couldn't. This reinforces your confidence and your abilities in general.

Tap the following areas as well, and reinforce yourself by saying the following:

Under the arms – I know I have what it takes to do this until the end.

Eyebrows – I no longer doubt myself and can envision how much better things will get after this.

Under the nose – My goal is right in front of me, and I'm getting there.

End the sequence by going back to the starting point again, with deep breaths in, and deep breaths out.

ATTAINING THE BALANCE – WEEK 3

It's the third and final week of your program, which means that you have practically mastered the art of EFT Tapping. At this point, your self-confidence has significantly improved, your stress levels and emotions are regulated and in check, and you have become more aware of your eating habits, thus improving your ability to discern. You may notice some changes in how you feel physically, thus the affirmation statement involved should be a recognition of your efforts and the results produced. "I can now see that I'm capable of more than I originally thought, and I'm loving it".

As you tap the inner point of your collarbone, congratulate yourself and acknowledge the effort you exerted and the mental strength it took for you to make it this far: I am a better version of myself now, and can do more and be more.

Breathe in the positive energy and the feeling of fulfillment, and breath out what's left of the negative energy. As you tap on other meridian points, focus on rewarding yourself:

- Your chin – I will no longer doubt myself because I am where I want to be.

- Karate chop – I feel better and will continue to feel better with the right mindset.
- At the top of my head – I have gotten this far thanks to my efforts, and I deserve to be here.

End the sequence by tapping the inner point of your collarbone as if patting yourself on the shoulder for the hard work you put into the program, feel the difference between where you were when you started and where you are now, and breathe in. Breathe out, and see just how far this change in mindset has taken you, despite the obstacles you had to brave to get here.

SAMPLE EFT SCRIPT FOR WEIGHT LOSS

SCRIPT 1- EVEN THOUGH I FEEL LIKE I CAN'T DO THIS...

1. Start tapping gently on the side of your hand (karate chop point).
2. Take a nice deep breath in and slowly out.
3. Repeat these 3 times – Breathe in and breathe out.
4. Continuing to tap on the side of the hand repeat the following --- Even though right now, I feel like I can't lose my excess weight. I feel like I just can't do this. I'm just going to put those feelings to one side and try something else.
5. Take a deep breath in and slowly breathe out, imagining the negative energy dissipating.
6. Shake out your arms.
7. Now, tap the side of your hand – Even though I've been feeling like I can't do this, deep down I know that's not true. Maybe I just need to shift my focus.
8. Now tap the following areas of the body…
9. Top of the head – Tapping out these negative feelings about being able to lose weight.

10. Start of the eyebrow – Shifting these feelings.
11. Side of the eye – Shifting the beliefs I have about losing weight.
12. Under the eye – Letting go of old, limiting ideas about weight loss.
13. Under the nose – These feelings that I can't do this.
14. Chin – This belief that I haven't got what it takes to lose this excess weight.
15. Collar bone – Tapping out any beliefs that are keeping me stuck.
16. Under the arm – Tapping out any beliefs that no longer serve me.
17. Move back to the side of your hand. Breathe in deeply and then breathe out.

SCRIPT 2 – I CAN DO THIS

TAP THE FOLLOWING AREAS…AND VERBALIZE

1. Top of the head – I am shifting my beliefs now so I can do this.
2. Start of the eyebrow – I'm shifting my beliefs to support me in losing this weight.
3. Side of the eye – I can do this.
4. Under the eye – I can lose this weight.
5. Under the nose – I can do this.
6. Chin – I'm starting to believe this is true now.
7. Collarbone – I can do this.
8. Under the arm – I'm starting to believe I can shift this excess weight.
9. Side of the hand – I can do this.

SCRIPT 3 – I CAN DO THIS (REPEAT)

TAP THE FOLLOWING AREAS… AND VERBALIZE

1. Top of the head – I can do this.
2. Start of the eyebrow – I can lose this weight.
3. Side of the eye – I can do this.
4. Under the eye – I can lose this weight now.
5. Under the nose – I can do this.
6. Chin – I'm now losing this excess weight.
7. Collarbone – I can do this.
8. Under the arm – I can do this.
9. Side of the hand – I can do this.
10. Breathe in – relax – Breathe out – Relax

Tips on how to customize the technique to fit individual needs

EFT tapping is a powerful technique that can be customized to fit individual needs, and when it comes to weight loss, women can benefit from tailoring their routines to address specific triggers and emotions.

Here are 10 tips on how to customize EFT tapping for weight loss, specifically tailored for women's individual needs:

1. Identify your specific triggers: Before commencing any EFT tapping program, it is vital to determine the particular triggers that contribute to harmful behaviors such as overeating or habitual bad behavior. This might be the result of tension, worry, boredom, or other

factors. You will be able to modify your EFT program such that it addresses the particular feelings you are experiencing once you have determined the causes of those feelings.

2. Create personalized affirmations: With EFT tapping for weight loss, affirmations are a powerful tool. But, it is essential to crafting individualized affirmations that speak to you on a particular level and meet the specific requirements of your life. Try saying something more particular, such as "I love and accept my body as it is," rather than expressing a general affirmation like "I am losing weight." For instance, you may try saying "I am losing weight."

3. Focus on self-acceptance: When it comes to weight loss, many women experience problems with their body image and self-esteem. Hence, if you want to get the most out of your EFT practice, including self-acceptance as a part of it may be quite useful. Reiterating uplifting statements to yourself and putting your attention on embracing yourself in the here and now are two great ways to improve your mental health.

4. Use visualizations: Visualizing yourself at your desired weight or engaging in healthy behaviors can be a powerful motivator during EFT tapping sessions. Try closing your eyes and imagining yourself feeling confident and healthy in your skin.

5. Target emotional eating: Emotional eating is a common issue for many women trying to lose weight. When creating an EFT tapping routine, focus on targeting the emotions that lead to emotional eating such as stress or anxiety.

6. Incorporate movement: Movement can help release tension and promote relaxation during an EFT session. Consider adding gentle stretches or yoga poses into your routine.

7. Experiment with different tapping points: While there are standard tapping points used in EFT routines, everyone's body is different and may respond better to certain points than others. Experiment with different points until you find what works best for you.

8. Practice regularly: Consistency is key when it comes to seeing results from EFT tapping for weight loss. Make sure to practice regularly - ideally daily - to see the maximum benefits.

9. Seek support from others: Losing weight can be challenging, but having a support system can make all the difference. Consider joining a support group or finding an accountability partner who also practices EFT tapping.

10. Be patient and kind to yourself: Weight loss is not always linear and progress may take time. Remember to be patient with yourself throughout the process and treat yourself with kindness and compassion along the way.

By tailoring an EFT tapping routine specifically towards their individual needs, women can see significant benefits not only in terms of weight loss but also overall mental health and well-being!

POTENTIAL CHALLENGES AND PRECAUTIONS

EFT tapping, also known as Emotional Freedom Techniques, is a form of alternative therapy that involves tapping on specific points on the body while focusing on negative emotions or thoughts. This technique has gained popularity in recent years as a potential tool for weight loss, but there are several challenges and limitations to consider when using EFT tapping for this purpose.

Lack of scientific evidence

One of the biggest challenges with using EFT tapping for weight loss is the lack of scientific evidence supporting its effectiveness. While some studies have suggested that EFT tapping can help reduce stress and anxiety, which may indirectly lead to weight loss, there is no conclusive evidence that directly links EFT tapping to weight loss.

Individual variability

Another challenge with using EFT tapping for weight loss is the individual variability in response. Some people may find that EFT tapping helps them manage their cravings and make healthier choices, while others may not experience any benefits at all. It's important to keep in mind that what works for one person may not work for another.

Limited research on long-term effects

While some studies have shown the short-term benefits of using EFT tapping for weight loss, there is limited research on the long-term effects. It's possible that any initial weight loss achieved through EFT tapping could be temporary if underlying emotional issues aren't addressed or if healthy lifestyle habits aren't maintained.

Not a substitute for medical treatment

EFT tapping should never be used as a substitute for medical treatment or advice from a healthcare professional. If an individual has an underlying medical condition contributing to their weight gains, such as thyroid disease or insulin resistance, they should seek appropriate medical care before relying solely on EFT tapping.

Need for consistency and commitment

Like any other form of therapy or behavior change, consistent practice and commitment are key to seeing results with EFT tapping for weight loss. It's important to tap regularly and consistently over time to see any potential benefits.

Potential psychological challenges

EFT tapping involves addressing negative emotions and thoughts related to food and body image, which can be challenging for individuals who struggle with disordered eating or body dysmorphia. It's important to approach this technique with caution and seek professional support if necessary.

In conclusion, while there are potential benefits of using EFT tapping as a tool for weight loss, there are also several challenges and limitations to consider. Lack of scientific evidence, individual variability in response, limited research on long-term effects, the need for consistency and commitment, potential psychological challenges, and the importance of seeking medical advice all highlight the importance of approaching this technique with caution and seeking professional support when necessary.

Conclusion

After delving further into the field of EFT tapping for weight loss, it is abundantly evident that this method has the potential to be an effective instrument for people who are wanting to drop unwanted pounds. Individuals can decrease stress and anxiety that may contribute to harmful behaviors such as overeating or unhealthy habits by tapping on certain meridian points while focusing on negative emotions or beliefs linked to food and body image.

There are still a lot of studies that need to be done on the effectiveness of EFT tapping for weight loss, however, a lot of practitioners and individuals have claimed that it works. It is crucial to note that this method should not be utilized as a single solution for weight reduction; rather, it should be used as a complementary practice along with other modifications to lead a healthier lifestyle, such as engaging in regular exercise and consuming a balanced diet.

Emotional Freedom Technique (EFT) tapping is one of the most popular forms of therapy since it can be practiced practically anywhere at any time and does not require any specialized training or equipment. In addition to this, the procedure is risk-free, does not include any sort of intrusive procedure, and has just a few minor adverse effects.

Emotional support and assistance in overcoming negative habits and attitudes around food and body image might potentially be gained by including EFT tapping into a weight reduction journey. In general. Before adopting any new approach to one's health and fitness, it is critical to discuss the plan with a qualified medical practitioner. Tapping with EFT has the potential to be an effective addition to one's toolset for weight loss if the individual is dedicated and consistent.

References and Helpful Links

Bach, D., Groesbeck, G., Stapleton, P., Sims, R., Blickheuser, K., & Church, D. (2019). Clinical eft (Emotional freedom techniques) improves multiple physiological markers of health. Journal of Evidence-Based Integrative Medicine, 24, 2515690X18823691.
https://doi.org/10.1177/2515690X18823691

Blacher, S. (2023). Emotional Freedom Technique (Eft): Tap to relieve stress and burnout. Journal of Interprofessional Education & Practice, 30, 100599. https://doi.org/10.1016/j.xjep.2023.100599

EFT tapping: The potential health benefits. (2022, November 8). EverydayHealth.Com. https://www.everydayhealth.com/wellness/how-to-use-standard-eft-tapping-plus-its-potential-health-benefits/

What is EFT tapping? 5-step technique for anxiety relief. (2017, December 1). Healthline. https://www.healthline.com/health/eft-tapping

What is EFT tapping? Evidence and how-to guide. (2019, September 26). https://www.medicalnewstoday.com/articles/326434